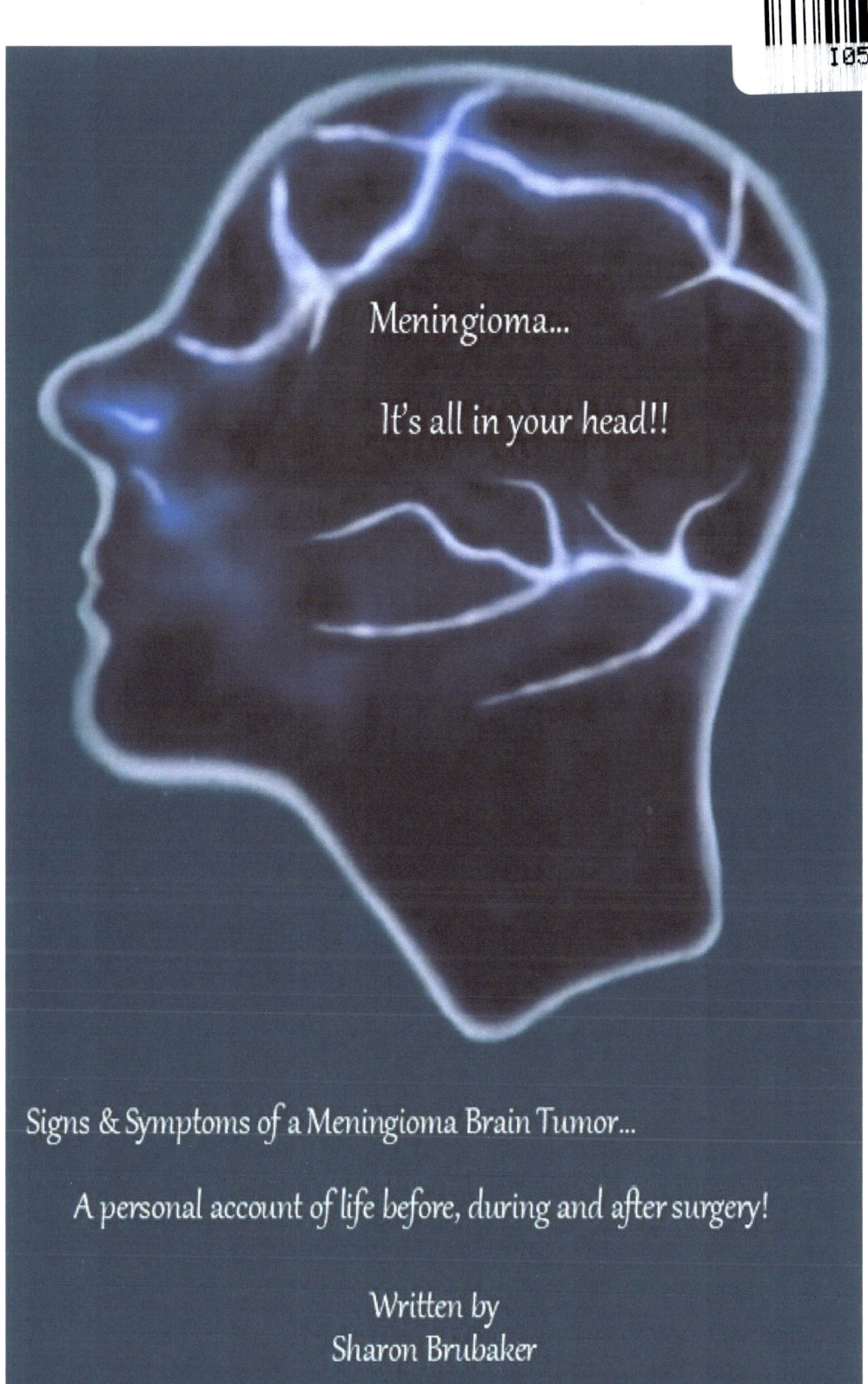

Designed by Sharon Brubaker

Introduction

You or someone you know has just been diagnosed with a type of brain tumor called a meningioma. "Don't let it scare you"! In the United States alone, meningioma tumors account for more than 37% of primary brain tumors. An estimated 34,210 people will be diagnosed with meningioma this year. Depending on the size and location, you will have several options. It will be monitored because it's small and currently stable or it needs to be removed.

Yes, it is a wake-up call, to hear those words you have a brain tumor. Believe me: it is ok. You will be surprised how much better you will feel once you learn more about this particular tumor. There are more than 120 types of brain and central nervous system (CNS) tumors. However, meningioma is the most common type of primary brain tumor.

I believe I had at least 95% of a large meningioma brain tumor removed on May 13, 2015. Five years later, each MRI completed has shown the tumor to remain the same size and stable. The first year, I had an MRI every six months, then once a year followed by every two years. Having shown no change, the next one will then be in five years.

With five years having past, I will share life before, during and after surgery, including any restrictions and time allotted for healing. Last, I want to ease your mind by sharing all of the exciting accomplishments I was able to achieve during this time.

Don't let anything stand in your way of being the best you can be. My life has been so much greater than it ever was before the tumor. I believe it is because I didn't appreciate what I was capable of doing or being. If you don't try anything new and different you can never say you failed. In your mind, you'll say it doesn't matter. But it does!

What if everything you tried out of the blue, you were successful at? What if all of a sudden one day everything made sense where it didn't before? I know one thing, the memory games described in this book made an amazing difference in life. It was as if my brain was charged. I remembered things I would normally have forgotten. Now it is clear, these games work for everyone not just for those who have had brain tumor surgery!

This book has been written for and is dedicated to every person in need of information, about meningioma brain tumors!!

Everyone who has been diagnosed with a meningioma brain tumor as well as information for family members and friends caring for someone who has one! I want to take away all of your fears, giving you as many answers you might need about surgery before, during and after.

This will also include information concerning meningioma tumors that would be monitored not removed. Don't fear or worry about something unknown.

My goal is to help you release any stress which will help the entire process travel a very smooth of all the surgeries I've had, this was not as major as you might think. I wouldn't be afraid if I had to have the same surgery again!

I have a very important list of Personal Dedications

The first dedication is to my **Lord and Savior, Jesus Christ**. I am a born again Christian, without Him, I wouldn't be where I am today, writing this book. I will look for His guidance so that I'm able to share my story and answer as many questions as possible.

I want to give a very warm, loving thank you to my son, **Stephen Brubaker** a young man who has not only been one of two of the greatest blessings in my life, he's always been there for me when I needed anything, he's my best friend. I never thought when he was born; he would be the first of many who would teach me the valuable lessons I would need in my life.

As parents, we try to teach them all of the lessons we've learned but looking back, he was the first one that came into my life and taught me; what life was seriously all about. Unlike his younger brother, he's on the quiet side but a very dedicated Christian. Knowing both of my sons would one day be in Heaven with me was the only thing that ever mattered, until grandchildren.

Stephen has one son, Tyler. Ben and his beautiful wife Andrea have three children. Andrew is newly married to Martyna. I want to mention Martyna has just published a wonderful book that you will find on Amazon called "Green Card Marriage" by, Martyna Nowacka. I have one grand daughter Julia. She blessed me with my first great-grandson King, who was born on my 60th birthday. Last on my list but never in my heart my grandson Luke. I always tell both of my sons how much I love them, how very proud I am of them and I'm their biggest fan! Now my grandchildren are in this same group!!

The next very warm and loving dedication is to my youngest son who has in so many ways become my hero, **Benjamin Brubaker**! I don't know anyone other than my two boys who know me inside and out! I always tried to be there for them if they needed to talk but never dreamt the day would come when the tables would turn. There were times after the brain surgery I felt like I was going to lose my mind and I couldn't have told you why just one of the side effects? I would call him and just start talking about everything that was bothering me. The next thing was uncontrollable crying. He has always been patient, a great listener, and knew exactly what so say. The last time this happened, he said Mom if you can calm down I would like to talk to you.

I agreed and what shocked me was everything he said to me sounded familiar. All of a sudden I remember saying to him, it looks like you were listening when you were growing up you!!!! He just laughed and said yes I heard everything you said, Mom. Never did I think he would bring my words right back to me, and in such a loving way! I mentioned to him not long ago it was as if his voice tone had changed, very soft, very mellow. We both said the same thing is was if the Lord was speaking through him.

One lesson for young parents reading this part, don't stop talking to your children just because you don't think they're listening, they're not only listening to every word but you are molding the life of someone who is part of you!! Not only did he remember our talks, but it is also the same way he raised his children. Not all children are like my Benjamin, there are times he reminds me so much of myself, very strong, outgoing, never afraid to try anything!

I guess he's the one I would have to say is definitely one of a kind because his door is open for anyone at anytime who needs to talk. He is an amazing Christian man who I love, respect, and he holds a very high place in my heart.

Another very warm and loving thank you is given to my best friend, who has deeply touched my heart! I have so much love, respect, and adoration for **Joel Freidhoff**. I always call him my rescue ranger! He's been there for me through the best and the worst of times for which there have been more health issues besides the tumor and he was always there along with his parents!

He has always given me the most love, understanding, strength, patience, guidance, and confidence anyone could ask for. Over the years I enjoyed watching a strict but loving father he's been with his two sons. Jonathan is his oldest and married to a beautiful young lady Meghan Sayers Freidhoff. She chose to be an RN for which I have a great deal of respect for her.

Both of her parents passed away from cancer right around the time she was married. I know she misses them so much wishing her little ones had her parents to spoil them! But Joel is trying to make it a little easier, he has a natural understanding when it comes to little ones and they love him!!

Christopher is his youngest son who also spoils the grandchildren; I know one day he too will make a wonderful father. For now, the one on one communication with them helps a lot!! Joel is excited along with grandsons, Charlie and Tommy. They were blessed with a little sister named Piper on October 14, 2020, at 5:45 am! Everyone is so excited!!

Another beautiful relationship Joel has is with his parents. He literally adores his Mother and Father, Walter and Patricia Freidhoff. I also enjoy listening to him talk about them. You can hear the love and respect for his two brothers Carl, Kurt, and his sister Laurie. I feel God has blessed me with some very warm, loving, people who all have a heart of gold and was always there when I was in need!

Every day Joel helps me strive to be a better version of myself. He is my inspiration, my mentor!! I love you are three words, it's the feelings deep inside that I've found speak in a higher volume He is my best friend, my confidant who I will be eternally grateful for!

The next dedication is a very warm thank you to an amazing surgeon who gave everything he could the day of and after my surgery; he seriously saved my life, **Dr. Brian Jankowitz**. Absolutely one of the most gifted neurosurgeons that I will be forever thankful for. I have also been blessed to have him since as a very dear friend.

Dr. Jankowitz has a genuine passion for what he does; his hands have been truly blessed by God to perform miracles. I'm one of many to prove this to be true. He believed in me, and has inspired me to reach higher levels than I ever thought possible like writing this book!

He planted the seed to do this book because of the way I excelled after my surgery at a higher level than most. There were times I would see him and he would say what's new. He loved hearing all of my accomplishments and encouraged me to continue. Then one time he said you should write a book. He even started it with me and did editing until he knew I couldn't walk away. He believed in me for which I will always Thank Dr. Brian Jankowitz for where I am today.

If anyone has been like a sister to me **Sandy Konsavich Getz** has!! She is my sister (in-law) and best friend. After the surgery, if I was alone and/or in need, she was always stopping by to check in on me, she took me to the store, always made sure I was doing everything right. After the surgery, she also endured my personality changes, they were not very pleasant at times but she took it all in stride and never became upset with me, she always left everything pass.

She was like an angel sent to keep an eye on me!! No matter what was going on in my life, all I ever had to do was call her; she was there for me and still is my rock I love dearly!!

Someone who I became very close to right after meeting her is **Judy Brubaker Cressley**. She's also my sister (in-law) and best friend. I've known her since 1975 and even with her brother and I divorcing, she never turned her back on me or judged me, she treated me with love, compassion, and understanding, she is not only a born again Christian that talks the talk but also does so in her walk.

She is someone that I could always count on. Years ago, we would go on long rails to trails walks, a time to talk, renew and relax. She has always encouraged and supported me. There were times over the years, we would talk for hours, sometimes we would cry, other times uncontrollable laughter. I cannot imagine my life without her; she has been such a strong mentor in my life as well as a sister. She is a great listener, tries to always be there when I need someone to turn to, someone I can trust. She has such a warm nature to her and a wonderful positive personality. She even helped edit this book, looking for mistakes with me!! Again, My Rock who I love dearly!!

Never, Ever Stop Dreaming!

When we hold our beliefs high, stay very focused and positive, we'll become and remain mentally aware. When we continue to look forward and focus on what is needed, our dreams become our reality. Why else would we hold onto a dream unless we wanted it to come true? With My Lord by my side and the Faith of that tiny mustard seed, anything is and has been possible.

All of my dreams have been granted one by one in my Lords' timing. I think some of the dreams in our hearts were placed there before we were ever born so we would look to Him for the answers needed in our life. Dreams come in all sizes and types of needs and desires. Whenever I need one to be granted, I will call upon the Lord, He hears my voice as soon as I call upon His name.

My experience has been, when I pray for a need or a miracle from deep within my heart, faith must, 100% must be applied; my voice is heard. When you no longer have any dreams left, life will feel very empty. Another reason I feel God places a few dreams in our hearts from the beginning. We need to stay focused on Him, hold our faith very strong and always keep looking forward.

Never Ever, Stop Dreaming! I've added this page to tell you how the brain tumor was actually my miracle. The reason I feel this way is that it changed my life in so many positive ways. There were times I felt frustrated but with the drive needed along with patience and faith I continuously progressed. Did the tumor keep me from learning and applying myself or was it a wake-up call?

Having memory problems after surgery, I craved knowledge in every area. I didn't even watch television without reading about the show. Don't let anyone limit your potential. One of two things, they could be worried about you or they have a competitive nature! When the latter half is true, do they ever ask themselves what has kept them from moving ahead?

We are personally responsible for what we accomplish in our life. Like many people, I'm at my highest level by just helping others. I try to find positive reasons for how I can get through my problems where most would find negativity. I refuse to let situations hold me back. I look at them as a way of helping at a higher level.

When you think about it, the hardships and severe challenges make us stronger and smarter only if we learn lessons from them. There are no more reading textbooks like we did growing up. Now we'll be the writer of our own book about our life. Will yours be a series or a best seller? Will your life be an inspiration to many or even one? It can be a new life, a more fulfilled life for anyone, brain surgery or not if you focus on what's important!

You can do anything you want if you just pick one dream at a time and take that first step forward! I've loved writing all my life but never thought I would ever actually have an opportunity to publish a book. This is a wonderful example of this page I just wrote. Pick a dream, and then move forward.

Sincerely Written In Christian Love & Faith

Sharon Brubaker

Contents

Introduction...2

Dedication to My Readers..4

My Personal Dedications 5

Never Ever Stop Dreaming! 10

In the beginning..14

MRI's and Reports..27

Meeting my surgeon..30

12 days later, relocated closer to home..37

Rebuilding life after surgery..47

Smule, singing promotes mental well being..50

Have you heard of Quora..51

Blessed with a Miracle..60

Important Questions & Answers..69

Questions to ask your doctor-neurosurgeon...76

Questions to ask about radiation..79

Sharon's Bios 80

Meningioma Website Links...84

The Mustard Seed Parable and Inspirational Thoughts..............................87

In the Beginning...

May 12, 2015 when I was diagnosed, I had no time to look for information as you are doing right now. I hope this book calms any fears you might be having. It includes my walk along with questions and answers. I've also included questions to ask your doctor before surgery. I've known people who have had brain tumors but no one that I could talk with.

This is why today, over 5 years since my surgery, I want to make this very easy for everyone to understand. I had many other health issues at the time; this was at a higher level to deal with but it still wasn't as bad as it sounds. The best way to start is to explain a little about what a meningioma brain tumor is.

A meningioma is a type of brain tumor that originates from the meninges, a thick membrane that covers the brain and spinal cord. These tumors are very slow-growing. 90% are benign and occur in the brain. Looking back, when I was in my early to mid-'30s, I remember having what seemed like serious migraine strength headaches.

I was given different medications, but nothing worked. Then after several months, I realized I wasn't having any more headaches. I thanked God they were gone. At the time, I never even thought a brain tumor could have been the reason I was having headaches that serious.

It stabilized which was a blessing; it gave me more time to catch up with technology in the medical world. Other than that, I felt I was doing very well I turned fifty. Then I was hit with one issue after another. I am sharing the other health issues so you will see how minor brain surgery was in comparison.

Dealing with only one issue can be trying but still it's only one issue. But to deal with one after another after another can not only be mentally trying but can take your body down physically as well. I was slowly getting more mentally tired; wandering each time something new came up would this be the last?

It was getting the best of me but I always had enough time to get enough strength to face the next challenge. And today proves you can make it through anything with a little perseverance! Please keep in mind none of these conditions had anything to do with the tumor; I just had to deal with each issue or condition one at a time.

Here is a list I was diagnosed with, within 10 years. I'm able to see things differently since I had the tumor surgery. More people fear going to the dentist, I can honestly tell you a meningioma is nothing to fear.

1. Total Hysterectomy
2. Spine Surgeries
3. Myxoid Cysts
4. Seizures
5. Epilepsy
6. Glaucoma
7. Meningioma Brain
8. Severe Dry Eyes

9. Conjunctival Eye Cysts   10 Spine Surgeries (3)

Over the next 5-year period I was diagnosed with:

1. Double Vision
2. Internal Hemorrhaging
3. Sepsis
4. Carpal Tunnel Surgery; both hands
5. Sinus Surgery (Twice, one year apart)
6. Deviated Septum Surgery
7. Gallbladder Surgery
8. Thyroid Biopsies for Cancer (Stable and cancer-free to date)
9. Vocal Cord, Throat Dysphasia

I also have been diagnosed with the following conditions that I deal with daily.

1. High Blood Pressure
2. Severe Acid Reflux
3. Glaucoma
4. Severe Dry Eyes
5. IBS Irritable bowel syndrome
6. Seborrhea Dermatitis
7. Arthritis

The first health issue I had to deal with after I turned 50 was a total hysterectomy, due to uterine fibroid tumors. After the surgery, my doctor told me there were more than could be counted. Because of that, he insisted on keeping everything that was removed and sending it all for cancer screening. Thank God, it all came back negative.

Uterine fibroids, also called leiomyomas or myomas, are non-cancerous growths that originate in the muscular wall of the uterus. Fibroids are the most common type of tumor found in female reproductive organs. It's hard to believe that many women with fibroids don't even have any symptoms.

You will see what I mean when you read the following signs/symptoms of uterine fibroids. When symptoms do occur, they can include any or all of the following:

1. Heavy and prolonged menstrual bleeding

2. Painful menstrual periods

3. Pressure and pain in the abdomen and lower back

4. Bloated and swollen abdomen

5. Frequent urination

6. Constipation

7. Pain during intercourse

Conditions two and three before the surgery were diagnosed at the same time. I had just met with a new ophthalmologist so she wanted to do every test because of my complaints. I had what looked like water blisters on both of my eyes. I was told I had dry eye, which made no sense to me because my eyes constantly watered. Since I always asked to be checked for glaucoma, that test was done also. The doctor was shocked at the reading.

My reading was 44; a normal reading is 12-22mm Hg. I was given drops for glaucoma called Latanoprost to start right away. Surgery was scheduled to remove the outside layer of both eyes because of the blisters. The surgery was done one eye at a time about 1 month apart. I also started using Restasis for the dry eye and they stopped watering. I will remain on Latanoprost and the Restasis for life because of these conditions.

Next on my list are 3 spine surgeries. I had several bad falls since I was in my thirties and had gone to a chiropractor regularly for several years. The day finally came when he said he could no longer treat me, I needed to see a surgeon. I knew I would hear those words one day. The first surgeon I saw said it would be too risky.

I could be paralyzed. I was beside myself because surgery or not it was becoming more and more difficult to walk. One day I was at work, the phone rang; it was my son Benjamin. He said; "Mom I think I found the answer to your back problem. I spoke with someone who went to a new place in Florida for surgery and he was completely happy.

He had no stitches, and only a few days of therapy right there at the facility. It was the newest spine surgery available. I'll give you the name, call them and see how you make out." I thanked him, looked them up online and called. To my surprise, a surgeon answered the phone. I explained my situation. He asked if I had a recent x-ray, I could fax him. I did and sent it to him.

Not 5 minutes later the phone rang. It was the surgeon. He looked it over and asked when I could get there. He had no problem explaining the details of the type of operation and basically that health issues would go away. I told him I would make the arrangements but it might be a week or two before I got there. He said, "No problem. You do not need an appointment for your surgery. You will receive an e-mail with the information needed for this procedure. Fill it out and have it with you when you arrive."

Over the next week, I completed all of the paperwork. I did what I needed to make the 7-day trip to have the surgery. I stayed with my Aunt Edie and Uncle Dick Shirk; he took me back and forth every day. He loved it. They always had such good food and he loved their coffee. It was nice spending so much time with him.

He told me some of the beautiful stories of how he met my aunt. My aunt passed away a short time ago and I know he is very lost without her; she was so full of energy and was simply an amazing woman. The spine surgeries I had were all done within a year and I have had absolutely no pain or problems with my back since.

Myxoid Cyst Surgery - a condition associated with osteoarthritis. It came on unexpectedly and then after a year or two it just went away. I had cysts that appeared on both hands near the fingernail. I kept having them surgically removed but they kept coming back. Finally, I had Joel machine me what looked like miniature dimes that it the area perfectly.

I placed them on and wrapped them with a material band-aid so they kept some pressure on them. They have never returned. An estimated 64 to 93 percent of people with osteoarthritis have Myxoid cysts. Twice as many women as men are affected. Seizures are a condition commonly caused by epilepsy. However, there are other reasons you could have a seizure, for example, a brain tumor. Since I still have a small tumor left, I will take anti-seizure medicine for life. This is why my records state I have epilepsy. There was a time five months after the surgery when my anti-seizure medicine had not been refilled and I had another comatose seizure.

When you have a seizure, you will lose your driver's license for six months. I had more than one type, but it started with a single seizure. I did not have them often; it might have been twice a month. I wasn't even sure of what was happening. I always licked my lips and made noises with my mouth, then smacked my lips seconds before a seizure.

Then I would get up and walk like a drunk and shake like I was being mildly shocked. I did not fall. I always kept moving but was unable to speak. These would only last a minute or two. Something else I noticed was I started sleeping 12 plus hours every night and would even fall asleep during the day. For me, it didn't make sense because I never slept more than 7 hours a night. I just functioned better with less sleep.

Once a seizure passed, I was exhausted. I felt very nauseated, dizzy and confused. I never had vision problems or headaches with these seizures.

They became scary because they got progressively worse. The next type I had is called a grand mal or status epilepticus. It repeats seizures, can, and will cause prolonged unconsciousness and coma.

I remember the first time I had one, May 11, 2015. There were no warning signs; I entered into a coma state. I would wake up sometimes for only seconds. I found a clock at one point and thought I need to look at the clock every time to keep track. I could still think clearly but was unable to speak. I still had no idea I was having another type of seizures. The first time to experience one of these, I was in the process of parking my car. If it had been a single seizure, I would have had the warning with my lips. But this was a first time experience with a comatose seizure.

I had no idea what was happening. I woke up to paramedics and police officers. Every time I woke up, they all started asking me questions. But I was unable to speak, I babbled. I remember looking at the clock. I was unconscious more than awake. Keeping track of the time was important to me. The next time I woke up it was after ten.

I had no idea they had already reached Joel and that he had already been in to see me because I had remained in a comatose state most of the time. Even when I woke up during this type of seizure I had little memory of being awake. Joel told me I was able to speak with him clearly; I just had no memory of him even being there. This type of seizure can seriously affect your memory.

The first time I woke up in the hospital after having a grand mal seizure, I still felt I was having seizures but no one diagnosed me with them and I was scared. With this type, my muscles would start to spasm and my breathing became shallow for a few minutes. I didn't feel like I was going to pass out I felt very numb and I then passed out. And what seemed to be the worst, one time when I woke up in the hospital I lost control of all bladder and bowel functions.

This had me sick with embarrassment. I still couldn't speak but never stayed awake for long. I remember one time waking up and I started throwing up. And still, if anyone was in the room with me they started asking me questions which I could understand, I had the right words in my mind to speak but could only babble. I felt that way all the time. It wasn't going to change, because I still had no memory of Joel being there.

This type of seizure can affect your mind and your short term memory in different ways. At this point, it was time to use my mind in a positive direction. A nurse came into my room to check my IV; I was lying on my left side, her back was right in front of me. Since I arrived, every time I woke up I looked at the clock and called out to the Lord. I said I need to be able to say two words, Father just two words, please help me.

I grabbed her by the back of her scrub, she turned to me and said are you ok? I shook my head no, I looked up towards the ceiling and took a deep breath then said the first of two words very clearly; brain. I had one more word to say and the confusion would be over. So I took another deep breath and said tume that was all I could say!

The nurse said do you have a brain tumor? I looked at her and shook my head yes! She ran out of my room yelling that I told her what I had. Several people came in and asked me the same question and I just kept shaking my head yes. One nurse said we are going to take you for an MRI of your brain to make sure. At this point with my symptoms, it had to make sense.

The next thing I knew I was back in a coma and didn't wake up until the next morning. Now that everyone knew what was causing all of my symptoms, everything fell right into place. It may sound strange but I know so many people who are reading this part, can agree you have experienced the same thing. It could have even been a time before caller ID; you would hear the phone ring and knew who called before you even picked it up. That is what a gut feeling or sixth sense feels like. After a period of time having little things like this happen you know to trust your thoughts! This is exactly what happened to me; how I knew I had a brain tumor. Always trust these feelings!

No doctor ever told me I had a brain tumor. This is how I diagnosed myself. When I told a doctor what was happening she thought I was having a mental break down or anxiety problems. She just didn't want to hear it. Funny thing, the comatose seizure that hit the hardest happened exactly 7 days after seeing her. Chalk it up to experiencing a sixth sense, gut feeling.

At first, you might have thought you were going crazy for having feelings like this. It's a feeling so deep within it doesn't go away; but at the same time, it gives you a peaceful feeling deep inside, an immediate understanding of what you need to do. Trusting your intuition is the ultimate act of trusting yourself. It will help you avoid unhealthy or dangerous situations.

I had a very strong gut feeling about the brain tumor. I knew I was right, some doctors don't want to hear you talk about your gut feeling. But mine was always right. May 12th. I was told I did have a brain tumor. To be honest, finally hearing those words I felt so relieved, I could breathe. They were in the process of transporting me to UPMC Mercy in Pittsburgh, Pennsylvania, for surgery.

I called to tell Joel I would be leaving soon; he was already told UPMC would contact him once the time of surgery was scheduled. There would be no reason for him to be there beforehand because of the tests they would need to run when I arrived.

He received the call and was told surgery was set for the following day, May 13, 2015, at 10 am I was finally on my way; I felt my stress drop drastically. My surgeon was present and waiting when we arrived, with surgery scheduled the next morning, he was ready to run every test needed right away.

One test that was given was an MRI with and without contrast. This contrast imaging test is a type of MRI that uses an injection of contrast dye. It's the best way to see the brain and spinal cord tumors, as well as any type of traumatic brain injury. It can also see multiple sclerosis, stroke, dementia, even infections.

Performing an MRI like this can sometimes allow doctors to tell if a tumor is or isn't cancer. Only hours away from surgery and it may be hard to believe but I am excited! I have that gut feeling everything will be just fine. The Lord has blessed me with one of the finest surgeons; I was in the best care now!

I had no fears, no worries. I just felt relieved I was now in the hands of someone who knew how to take care of me. Now I can take a deep breath and seriously just get some rest.

MRI's and Reports

Meningioma Photo

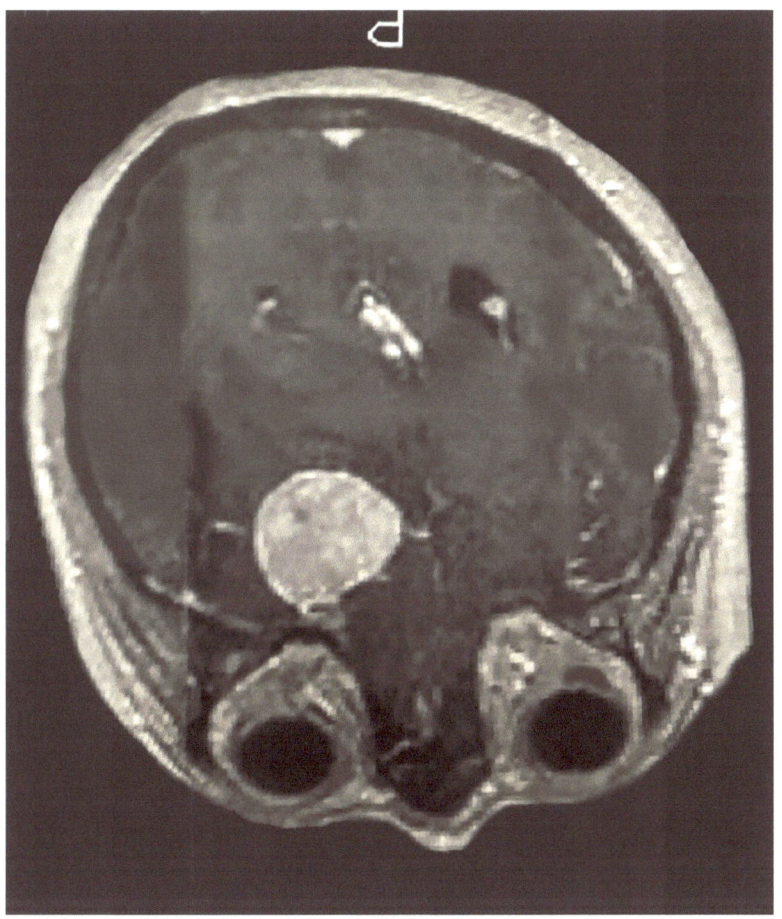

Here is a photo of my meningioma tumor, which is right behind the left eye along with my first MRI report…My Meningioma brain tumor was measured at 2.9 x 3.1x 3.6 cm. I've talked with others who have not only multiple tumors but one or two people had a tumor that measured as high as 6 cm. Most meningiomas are known to be noncancerous. Cancerous meningiomas make up a little more than 1% of all primary brain tumors. The percent means how many out of 100.

May 12, 2015 Meningioma Brain Tumor MRI Report

CLINICAL HISTORY:
Left basal ganglia mass from OSH; PLEASE PERFORM WITH STRYKER PROTOCOL/IMAGE GUIDANCE

COMPARISON:
None.

TECHNIQUE:
Multiplanar multisequence MRI of the brain emphasizing short and long TR contrast information with axial diffusion multiplanar postcontrast imaging. The patient was administered 18 cc of IV MultiHance.

FINDINGS:
There is a large parenchymal lesion seen which appears extra-axial and demonstrates broad dural base along the medial aspect of the greater wing of sphenoid, overlying region of cavernous sinus, anterior clinoid and extending medially to the left aspect of the sella and extending anteriorly over the posterior aspect of the roof of the orbit. The lesion measures 2.9 x 3.1 x 3.6 cm and demonstrates avid enhancement. There is considerable mass effect related to the lesion with extensive vasogenic appearing edema in the left frontal lobe and throughout the left basal ganglia. There is asymmetric effacement of the left lateral ventricle with 13 mm of left to right midline shift. There are a few small cystic or cleft-like areas of CSF at the margin of the lesion as well. The imaging appearance is most consistent with a meningioma.

There is no restricted diffusion or evidence of acute infarct. The intracranial flow voids appear preserved. The supraclinoid component of the left ICA may be partially encased by the lesion. The carotid terminus, proximal left A1 and M1 segments are displaced posteriorly by the lesion. Correlation with concurrently performed CT angiogram advised. No additional lesions are seen.

No additional parenchymal enhancement is noted.

Impression

IMPRESSION: 2.9 x 3.1 x 3.6 cm extra-axial avidly enhancing mass lesion at the anterior clinoid on the left causing mass effect and severe edema which is most consistent with meningioma. The lesion appears to encase portions of the supraclinoid carotid artery on the left and displace the proximal A1 and M1 segments posteriorly. 11:00 PM 05/12/2015.

Meeting My Surgeon...

I remember my surgeon introducing himself to me the afternoon I arrived, but I don't remember being awake at all after that which was fine with me. About a month or two before the tumor was found, I slept at least 12 plus hours every day! This was strange because just about all my adult life I had problems sleeping.

I remember waking up that morning in the operating room, thinking not only how bright it was but how many busy people were in the room. I just laid there watching them. The surgeon Dr. Brian Jankowitz came to me introduced himself and said I need to talk with you for a few minutes. He asked me my name I told him. He asked me if I knew why I was there;

I told him I knew I had a brain tumor that he would take care of for me. He said I do have to tell you it's common for the heart to stop beating at least once, there is a 50/50 chance you may not make it, but I am not worried, I know you'll be just fine! He had such a happy look on his handsome face and I could hear the strength and confidence in his voice.

I wasn't worried at all, I was happy to finally be right where I was. I didn't see it as an end but as a beginning. Then he said you must not be worried because your blood pressure is normal, which is very unusual. I told him I wasn't worried at all.

He said you also seem to be thinking very clearly. He then asked if I had any questions for him. I said, yes, did you get a good night's sleep, which made him laugh. I took him off guard, which was a good thing. I then asked him are you feeling well this morning. He smiled and said yes, I slept well and feel great, no one has ever asked me that before surgery, thank you.

He said is there anything else? I said I do have something to tell you. If I die and you have a hard time getting my heart to beat, please don't feel bad or worry about it, it's not in your hands it is just my time to go home. I am a born again Christian and I'm not afraid to die because I know I will be in heaven. Seriously, it's ok. I don't want you feeling bad about it, I'll be very happy to be home.

If it is not my time and it gets to be, too much for you God will send someone to help you. Dr. Jankowitz smiled and said well, this is only going to be about a 4 to 5-hour operation, you will be ok and other surgeons are not in the habit of just coming in like that to help, but it is a nice thought. He said do you have anything else you want to say I have to get ready.

I said I guess just good luck!! He laughed and I thought it's so nice to put a smile on the face of the doctor that is going to be doing such serious surgery. Either way, I wasn't worried. He no sooner left and I don't remember a thing until I woke up in my room. And I honestly can't tell you how long after surgery I woke up; did they wake me up shortly after?

I know the surgery started around 10:30-11:00 am and was not finished until around 2:00 am so it took a little longer than 4-5 hours for a reason. After the surgery was over Brian sat down and talked with Joel, told him how everything went, that he was happy with how well I did. He asked Joel if he wanted to see me before he. Yes, he was happy to hear that. Joel told me he walked into the room, over to me and held my hand. After a few minutes, he headed home. The next day after work, he came right back down to see me and did so every day that left followed until I was released which was twelve days total.

Unfortunately, for the first three days, I was unconscious more than I was awake. And because of the alarms, I set off when I moved, the nurse showed Joel how to reposition the drainage tubes coming out of my head. I can say with total accuracy when I did come around, I had zero pain or discomfort of any kind. The drain tubes in my head and the IV made it a little uncomfortable so I did have to take it easy.

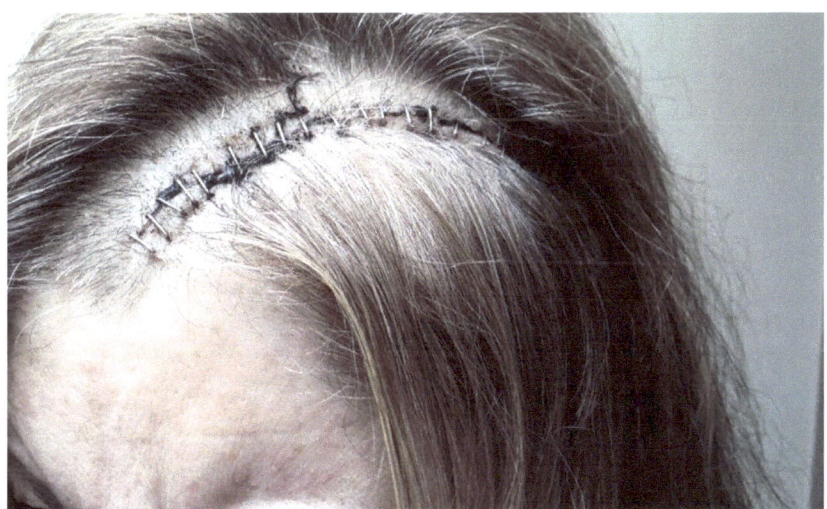

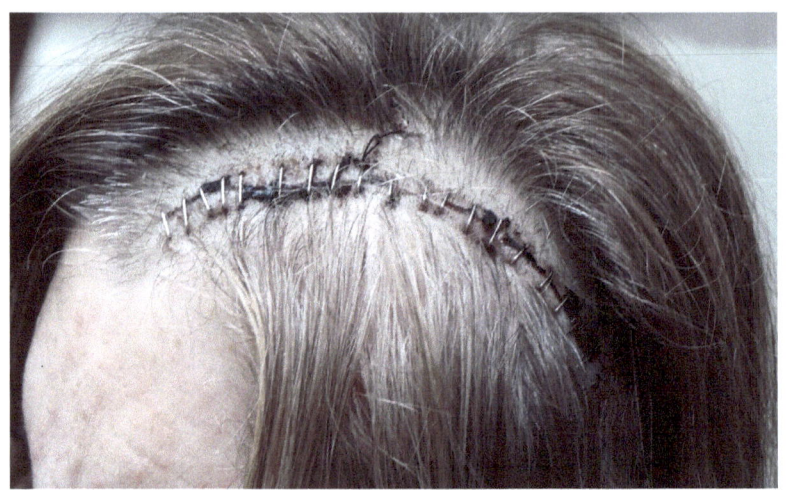

These photos don't really need an explanation…

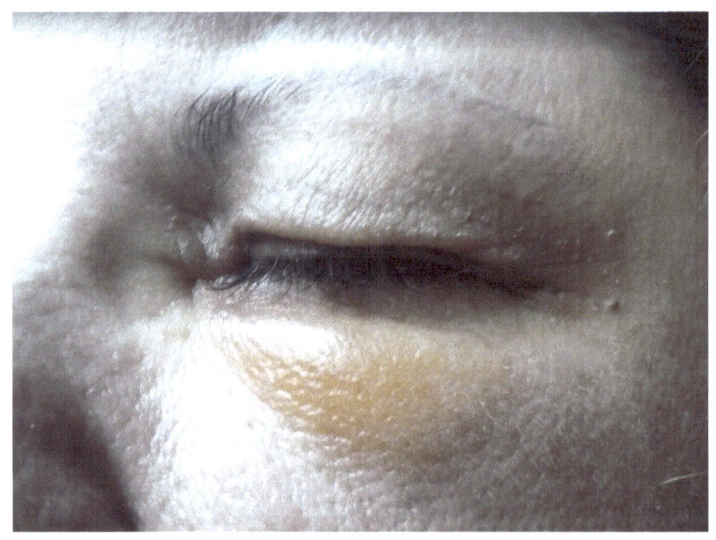

I had to ask, how many staples did you put in my head? He said 39, I said geeeeze couldn't you have found a place to put one more in to make an even number? He laughed, looked at the nurse and said, we've got one of those, go get my staple gun so I can put one more in. I wanted to see him laugh again; I didn't care how many staples were in my head.

To this day I think of the stress he was under doing that surgery, I will always think about it and be grateful for being put in his care!
Here I am, a little over five years later the tumor is still about the size of a grape and has remained stable, everything he did was a good call at the time. In the first few days he stopped by with another doctor, a friend of his that just happened to be checking on one of his patients the night of my surgery and saw Brian in the operating room.

He opened the door and said this isn't the same one from this morning, is it? Brian said yes, he said I'll wash up and be in. Does God work in mysterious ways? Joel was there every day which helped me heal so much faster. I always loved waking up, seeing his handsome face which always had a big smile then he would softly say Hi. My heart would skip a beat, he's been my best friend from the day we met, I don't know where I would be without him, He's always been there for me through the good and the bad times and unfortunately, there have been more bad health times than good.

He went through allot and never complained, he always encourages me to feel better to be optimistic and always tells me how proud he is of me. I've thought so often about how he sat in the waiting room while I was in surgery. It had to be so mentally stressful for him, he's never complained. Then I thought about my surgeon Brian, how he was on his feet the whole time. I thought he had to have a backache!! It's not just a job for doctors like Brian Jankowitz; it's his passion that saves people's lives.

He never gives up because every tumor is different and can be a learning experience. Something very unusual happened at my sixth month MRI and check up. Brian even said, don't ask me any questions because it's the first time I've ever seen anything like this. When I went in for my six-month MRI & checkup, my doctor said I have good news, and no bad news but odd news.

He said the good news is, the swelling in the brain went down completely and your tumor is stable everything looks fine. The odd news is when the swelling went down, your brain sort of shrunk; the front left quarter of your skull is empty. He said he has never seen this before so he couldn't answer any questions. He was slightly confused but at the same time happy to see how far I progressed mentally and physically.

I also had double vision after the surgery and was sent to see an eye surgeon at the same hospital who told me after reading my records that I had glaucoma for 15 years prior to it having been diagnosed. He asked me if I had ever been tested for glaucoma and I told him I always asked to be tested because my grandmother had it. Always having a gut feeling, I felt I had it also. I then asked him how he knew this.

He said over half of the back of your left eye is deteriorated. He said you should be blind in that eye, I can't understand how you can see. I said I'm proof God exists!

What happens down the road after surgery depends on the tumor size, location, and timing of the surgery but seriously your attitude more than anything. In my situation the brain was extremely swollen, this tumor had to be removed. If it had been even a few weeks earlier, it might have made it a little easier. After twelve days in the hospital, I'll now be moved to a rehabilitation facility very close to home. It was nice knowing I'll be starting different types of therapy and Joel will not have to drive to Pittsburgh every day.

12 days later, relocated closer to home...

After I was settled in the facility close to home, one woman came to see me tell me what all to expect. I kept quiet and just listened to her because I had to evaluate what she was saying and see if this was true. One thing remained strong that was my stubbornness! I did things to the beat of my own drum not someone else's!

And in this case I knew me, did I have the drive and the patience needed to pick up the pace in my recovery? I was told I could be there for three or four months. As soon as I heard that I remember thinking, I don't think so!! As the days of therapy passed they had plans of keeping it in slow-motion. I wanted them to pick up the pace, I wanted to go home. They felt the level they were doing therapy was in my best interest. They didn't want me to do anything without supervision.

I understand that to a point but if I have to go to the restroom and call for someone and they don't come within a certain period of time I need them to be there, guess what? I'm getting out of bed and going myself and yes I got yelled at several times but it didn't get them there any faster and it didn't keep me from going by myself. It was the same with showering, the first day there was a very nice nurse there to help me and it worked out great.

I had a chair I sat on, took my shower, I washed my hair, no problem. After the first day, everyone was busy or didn't respond so I got my things together and went in sat down on the chair and took my shower. Someone always came in to check on me.

It got to where they would say there's no point in arguing with you, you're going to do whatever you want to whether we like it or not! I said don't take it personally; I have to do things in the way I feel it needs to be done. I just need to pick up the pace. I had a little bit of a difficult time walking independently and realized I could get hurt if I wasn't careful.

I took walks down the halls as often as I could and held on to the bar along the wall. Everyone saw that I was trying as well as being very careful, it also allowed me to advance more than if I would have waited for a therapist.
I just couldn't imagine being there for three or four months, I knew I would be more comfortable at home. I made notes on the types of therapy I was having every day so I could continue them when I was home and did. Having been there only a week, one of the therapists came in to see me and said they all had a meeting and decided I could go home on Friday. YES, I did everything right. I knew I would continue to excel at home with a comfort level you only have when you are at home.

They did send someone to check in on me to see if I needed help, someone, to cook, clean, help with showering. When the woman arrived I was folding clothes, my home was very clean as it should be I live alone. She looked around and couldn't believe that between three and four weeks prior, I had major brain surgery. She looked at Joel and said, she doesn't need anyone, for anything, she's doing great.

He agreed I was taking very good care of myself and told her what all how he was doing for me every day. Joel had all of my daily pills in order with the times marked when they should be taken as well as always made sure I had lunch and or dinner, whatever I wanted because he didn't want me to cook. He checked on me constantly. I remember when I was released from Pittsburgh to come back home, Brian had a talk with me telling me what I could and couldn't do, what I could expect and not to worry about anything else. I remember him telling me I would not be walking and talking at 100% for possibly months and that was ok, he said just relax, rest. I was surprised how right he was on everything he said but it bothered me.

I wanted to get back to normal life as quickly as possible. I had already put the surgery behind me as if it never even happened or it was just no big deal, but I guess it was, and every day I looked in the mirror and saw those staples, it was another reminder of just how serious it was. They were removed the first week in June.

The one thing I was thankful for was Brian only shaved a line of about an inch wide where he was going to cut. He said he did that so when the staples were removed I could fix my hair and not be reminded of it. And he was right; it was very easy to forget it ever happened. I never had pain any kind after the surgery, not even a headache!

Once you have had a seizure, you will lose your driver's license for six months; and you can't get it back unless you've gone six months seizure-free. The third Saturday in June, I was bored, it was five weeks after surgery and the staples were gone so I decided I would go for a walk. I made sure my cell phone was fully charged; I had a full cold bottle of water to drink and was wearing comfortable shoes.

The temperature was in the mid-'70s; it was an absolutely beautiful day, to say the least! One thing I realized that day, you can drive an area for years and miss so much along the way. I decided to go for a walk and take my time. I wanted to take the time to stop and seriously smell the flowers, to enjoy some of the little spots along the way.

I left my house around twelve and headed up towards Joel's place, which was uphill the whole way. One of the first stops I made was to stand on the bridge and look out over a multi-line train track. I have always loved trains, so it was interesting to watch the activity. From where I started it was all uphill, at first, it took the wind out of me a bit but I hit an area where I started a nice steady pace.

Years ago, my sister in law Judy Cressley and I would walk the rails to trails as much as we could. She loved looking for familiar flowers and brought things to my attention that I would have missed. So today walking alone, I thought about her and took a closer look at things not wanting to miss anything. A little way into my hike, I was lucky enough to see a small turtle so I picked it up and put it over the side of the hill away from the road.

Continuing seemed like it was going faster than I expected. The next thing I knew I was at my destination. I crossed the road to start back Freidhoff Lane where I saw a big blue truck owned by Joel's brother Kurt headed out the road. But who by chance today was driving it? Joel. He stopped beside me and said tell me someone just gave you a ride!

I said no looking at my watch again; I said I walked up two and a half miles in just under 3 hours, I was so happy and in need of a glass of water. He was soon back and told me I was not allowed to walk home. I asked him why it would be so much easier than the walk I just had uphill. He said you could have been killed walking that road.

I said I would have never done it if I had any fear; there was plenty of room on the one side, that I felt safe. He said, either way, when you go back for another MRI you can be upset with me but I am going to tell your doctor about this walk today. I said whatever. He said you could have something wrong because of the surgery; we have to tell your doctors everything.

There was nothing I could do to stop him; he was taking care of me I couldn't complain. Five months later when I saw my surgeon, Joel told him the story after the initial visit, he asked for the description of the road again. Dr. Jankowitz asked me if I did walk that and I said with excitement in my voice yes, I walked 3 miles in, then said I'm sorry I won't do it again.

He said don't apologize, I'm surprised and proud of you. He said I never would have expected to hear this! Keep up the good work but please do be careful! I was on more pills than I had ever been but it wasn't just because of the brain surgery had fibromyalgia and other conditions mentioned earlier that I was still being treated for. I think the only pill added was an anti seizer pill called Keppra, I was on more pills than I had ever been but it wasn't just because of the brain surgery had fibromyalgia and other conditions mentioned earlier that I was still being treated for.

I think the only pill added was an anti seizer pill called Keppra, then Zoloft. If I remember correctly I still have a tumor about the size of a pea left; I'll remain on Keppra for life. With that being said I would still have a seizure if I didn't take Keppra every day. Brian sent that prescription to my family doctor and no one knows what happened but I didn't have that pill to take and at the end of October I had another grand mal seizure at night while I was sleeping. Having wandered seriously would I ever have another seizure?

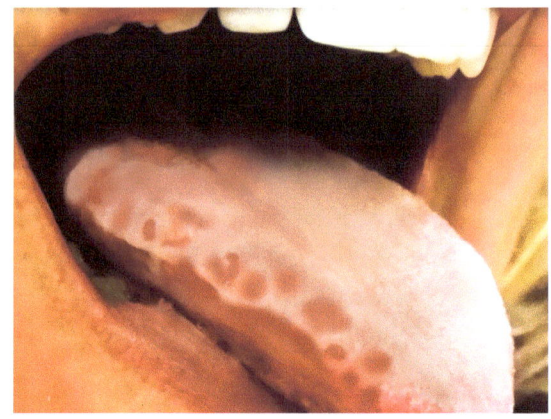

Yes I did but I didn't know why! This is a photo I showed Brian where he diagnosed another grand mal seizer. When I woke up I didn't know what was wrong except my tongue hurt so bad when I looked in the mirror, my teeth's imprint was embedded all around my tongue. Knowing I had an appointment with Brian in two weeks I took a few pictures with my cell phone and decided to show him and ask him what he thought. Before every doctor visit I always put every prescription bottle I took every day into a bag and took it with me to my appointments.

It made everything so much easier and the doctors' office liked it as well!! My memory was so bad; this is why I put every pill bottle in a bag to take with me! They would double-check it with their list. It made it so much easier for both of us. So I showed Brian the photos of my tongue and he shocked me when he immediately said you had another seizure! Why aren't you taking your anti-seizure pill? I said I don't know and I honestly didn't know. I gave him my bag. After he finished looking through all of the bottles, he looked at me and said, there are no bottles here for Keppra. You had another seizure, your six months waiting period to get your drivers' license is only a few weeks from being complete and now because of this seizure, it will have to be recorded and you'll have to start a six month waiting period all over again. He said he sent the script to my doctor and couldn't figure out what happened but told me I have to keep track of what I need to be taking every day and make sure I take them "every day"!! It's extremely important; I will be on an anti-seizure pill for life. It's because I still have a brain tumor even though it is very small.

It's still large enough and or located in an area where I will continue to have seizures if I don't take Keppra every day! I was also diagnosed with Epilepsy because of the seizures. I'm not happy but there's nothing I can do about it. When you have a condition that causes seizures you are diagnosed with epilepsy.

Page 1 2019 Meningioma Brain Tumor MRI Report

The first year or two after surgery, I had an MRI every six months. The tumor has remained stable in size with no other types of complications. I was then checked on a yearly basis still having an MRI with and without contrast. The last one I had was in May of 2019. This is the report from that test.

HISTORY: 60-year-old female with a history of left pterional Craniotomy and resection of skull base meningioma in 2015. Follow-up examination.

TECHNIQUE: Multiplanar multisequence MRI of the brain emphasizing short and long TR contrast, with axial diffusion, ADC and EADC maps. Multiplanar post contrast imaging was performed following uneventful administration of 20 cc MultiHance intravenous contrast without documented reaction.

COMPARISON: MRIs of the brain dating back to 11/20/2015, the most recent of which is about 11/14/2017.

FINDINGS:
There are operative changes from prior left pterional craniotomy and meningioma resection. There is associated encephalomalacia in the left frontal and anterior left temporal lobe, unchanged from prior. Stable subcortical T2/FLAIR signal seen at the site of resection reflect gliosis. No additional new abnormal focal parenchymal T2/FLAIR signal is evident.

A 0.7 x 1.2 cm enhancing mass centered at the left anterior clinoid process (series 11, image 19) is not significant changed since the prior exam of 11/14/2017. The mass encases the left supraclinoid internal carotid artery by roughly 50% without significant narrowing. It also abuts the left A1 segment of the left ACA and left optic nerve posteriorly, also unchanged from prior. All major intracranial flow voids are preserved. No new enhancing masses are evident. There is linear enhancement in the region of the right internal auditory canal with extension to the labyrinthine and geniculate segments of the right facial nerve canal, similar to the prior which may be vascular in etiology.

The ventricles are stable in caliber and configuration. The basal cisterns are preserved. There is no acute intracranial hemorrhage, mass effect or midline shift. Scattered areas of susceptibility seen along the resection cavity reflect remote blood products.

Visualized orbits and globes are unremarkable. A mucosal retention cyst is seen within the right maxillary sinus with trace mucosal thickening in the left maxillary and sphenoid sinuses. The mastoid air cells are clear.

Impression

Residual meningioma along the left anterior clinoid process abutting the left carotid terminus, left anterior cerebral artery A1 segment, and left optic nerve, unchanged since prior exam of 11/14/2017. 2. No new enhancing mass lesion or acute interval change from prior. 3. Linear enhancement extending from the right internal auditory canal into the labyrinthine and geniculate segments of the right facial nerve canal, similar to prior may be vascular in etiology, but correlation for right facial nerve symptomatology is recommended.

5/8/2019 2:09 PM

Rebuilding your life after brain surgery

A few things I've learned over the years, is to stop closing doors on things I want to do. How do you know if you can or can't do something if you've never even tried? To be honest one of the best things that can happen from the surgery is serious memory problems. Yes, memory loss can be frustrating in some ways but I saw answers not problems, I was determined to use it to benefit my life in some way.

When I learned how my memory was affected; I wasn't exactly sure what I could or couldn't do before the surgery. In a way I now had the eyes of a child, I could do anything. So anything that looked like fun or interesting I tried. One thing I want to say; nothing you read will be written out of pride. Everything I set out to do was for a desire to learn or simply for fun!

What I want is for this to light a fire within you. I don't want you to have a brain tumor or memory problems to live before you die! Everyone has gifts or talents they are unaware of that could change your life or someone else's. With everyone's busy work schedule, raising our family, trying to take care of everyone in our life, we always forget ourselves.

Believe me, once you do something and see with your eyes, feel with your heart how you've changed, helped or maybe even saved someone's life, you'll no longer walk you'll run. You will want to do everything you can to continue this new road you're on because going with your gut eling, your sixth sense…you'll change the world around you with each step you take.

I have is a keyboard with a large external amp. Joel would play when he came to visit. When he became very busy at work, I no longer heard the music and missed it. One day I thought why not try to play something myself. I sat down I turned it on along with the amp and just started playing the keys. Before long I started to hear notes of songs I knew.

I sat and played by ear and within an hour I could play a song from start to finish. I loved it. One evening I was playing a Christmas song when he walked in. I asked him if he recognized the song, he said yes, but you're missing a note here and there.

He came over to me and said go ahead and start again. I played with one hand, He went over to the piano and brought over a book, opened it to the page of the song I was playing, and told me to try it again. I started to play, he said wait a minute, read the music, and I said I don't know how to read music. He said you can't read music; you play one-handed and can play just about as well as I can.

You need to learn to read music that would help. I said Stevie Wonder can't read music, he smiled and said the good call never mind. Something to think about is to find something that relieves stress on bad days, an outlet. Brain surgery or no brain surgery everyone needs an outlet! I found besides playing the keyboard I enjoy all types of crafts, being creative.

Smule, singing promotes mental well being!!

A favorite of mine has always been singing and recording music. I don't come close to the voices you'll hear on the radio it's just a personal mental stress release for me. No matter what your problem, occasion or mood you're feeling, you'll find a number of songs written all about it!

Here's what music does to your brain. Sound drifts through your auditory pathways, the pitch registers in your mind, rhythm rocks through the motor regions of your brain, your brain figures out the tune, connects it to your memory and then decides if you want to sing it! Music lights your brain up!!

If you want a wonderful app to try it's one I've fallen in love with called Smule! I've even been able to upload some of the songs to my Youtube page which I would love anyone reading this to subscribe to. My son Benjamin has a very successful Youtube page all about rc cars and trucks called "Buy it Break it Fix it"! Listen, rc cars and trucks are owned by allot of women today too!! Check out his page if you can, the companies behind these products do some amazing give always! He's also tried to talk me into starting some type of forum where I would talk about my life, health issues, and everyday life then allowing my followers to join me live and ask questions. This might be my next step to follow, it would not only be very fulfilling but I love people it would be allot of fun! Join Smule, look for me and we'll move forward together!

Have you heard of Quora?

After the surgery, I was literally starving for knowledge and this is when it occurred to me how much of my memory had been seriously affected. So I read everything I could. I would look up biographies to read about people I watched on television. About a year and a half after the surgery out of the blue, I received a call from a friend of mine from high school, David Solt.

David saw my Facebook posts about my surgery. He said he understood what I was going through and thought I might enjoy helping others by answering questions for people about the tumor I had. Having not talked with him in so many years I'll never forget how he talked to me in a way that made me feel like it was a done deal, he gave me the confidence he thought I needed!

David said all I would have to do is join a website called Quora; I could help anyone on this website who either has a meningioma tumor or knows someone that does. I would receive an email asking if I could write an answer or pass. It allows you to answer questions on a personal level of experience, which can be very nice for both parties.

This seemed like such a positive way to help with such important decisions and conditions. I joined the international website that answers every type of question you can think of. If you haven't heard of this web site, please read about it on Wikipedia, I know once you start reading, it's like a good book you just can't stop!

You can answer questions on any topic you know about or conditions you have had, via a personal level, or you can do research for people looking for answers. I checked meningioma brain tumors, fibromyalgia, glaucoma, severe dry eyes, Salvation, Christianity, and a few other things.

I received so many awesome questions every day. With that being said, most of them I did research to answer them if I had no personal experience. It was a huge learning experience for me, which was exactly the direction I needed to move into. The second day I answered a question about brain surgery and one person came back stating a reply having had surgery like yours, they had to let you die then bring you back to life after.

I replied why that wasn't true and had other people posted the same reasoning I did. That surprised me was the next day I received an email from the website asking me to take the link they sent me and make the corrections to the answer I had given. I immediately thought I was in trouble. But once I was on that page and started reading the highlighted areas, they had for correction; it was spell check and commas, semicolons, which had been edited.

I replied telling them I had made all of the corrections then commented, I never expected to have spell check done because of how many people were writing daily on their web site world wide!! Quora is a privately owned, "ad free" website. Ad free is the best they could have done, no pop ups of any kind!! World wide there are approximately 400 million monthly users, 40 million users in the US alone.

Answers are given on over 400,000 different topics. The estimated valuation is 2 billion with 722 employees worldwide. Does wow even cover these numbers? This one web site will greatly educate anyone who has the time. I was then asked if I noticed how many people read my answer. I was then told where to look for that information and all of the feedback I had received.

I went back, looked, and again thought I have to be wrong. It overwhelmed me, in two to three hours over 700,000 people worldwide read my answer, over 2K people gave me thumbs up. So many commented with their own stories which I loved reading. I had so many people post a reply to that one question that I answered within 48 hours, if I added that one question with the replies, it would add 64 pages to this book. I would love it if you went to the website to read it.

In November 2012, Quora introduced what was called Top Writers Program. It was how they recognized individuals who contributed valuable content to the site. About 150 writers are chosen each year. Top writers are invited to occasional exclusive events and received gifts such as branded clothing items and books. Joining isn't mandatory to read unlimited questions & answers about everything you can think of.

You can even search for a question or topic and it will bring up all that was asked from the past. I was then told they don't do a spell check on every answer only the ones that would be published in the next book. I honestly felt as if I would wake up and say that was some dream!

It seriously took time for me to comprehend this because I was doing something I not only enjoyed but it was educating me, which I needed. Then one day I received an email congratulating me on being named Quora Top Writer for 2018, for "Excellence in Writing". It's funny but I was so used to doing a certain amount of research to answer questions; I had to find out what this was all about because I never heard of it or took notice to it before. I replied and asked what it was all about.

They explained how I answer questions in a way that anyone can understand no matter what their intellectual level is. When people are writing to you asking about serious problems and conditions, you have to write an answer that could possibly save a life!! What they wrote me back touched me deeply; I felt needed and knew I was doing everything right. I always felt I was giving all I had but this in its own way said job well done.

I want to give a very special, personal thank you here to David Solt who reached out to me with something he thought I might enjoy doing but didn't realize how important it would one day be to me. Many people only think about doing or saying something. It means nothing until you do it not just think it. David didn't think about it, he called me and it's because of that one call he made that day, it has helped me to get to where I am today not only with Quora's website but also with this book.

Don't just think about something whether it is for you or someone else, do it!! Trust me you won't be sorry, lives are changed everyday by action, by doing not by remaining mentally and/or physically sedentary or quiet!! I want to also thank Quora for allowing me to add them to my book. You've helped me grow, and educated me in such an amazing way, not to mention I've made so many friends a few who actually was in serious need of brain surgery for a meningioma brain tumor.

Having written back and forth, the surgeries were done and their life was saved. I couldn't have helped anyone without this website for which I will be forever grateful. If you haven't seen or heard of this webpage called QUORA, please check them out on Wikipedia. Then go to Quora's webpage and look up some questions you might have had for sometime but no where to find the answers.

I don't think there's been a question that hasn't been asked on their website yet! Here's an example, did you ever think anyone on earth has sued God? Sued God and won? How could anyone win a lawsuit against God? Go to their web page, do a search and enjoy reading. If you have something you believe could help someone, please join it's free.

Another addition is the greater number of people read your questions and/or answers you will be paid!! Take the time to help anyone you can, trust me you won't be sorry!! I actually read not long ago that Quora is right at the top with Google and Wikipedia for being a top informational resource. Wikipedia is another website I belong to and love. Wikipedia has the complete history of Quora, which is nice reading.

Here's something that might make you laugh aloud because it sill makes me! Something happened one day and I had no idea what was happening or even how to try to explain it. I kept having strange feelings in my face and would be lightly gasping for breath.

My nose would tingle and feel itchy along with my eyes. It scared me. Every time I felt this strange sensation, I would do anything I could think of to stop it. I felt something bad would happen. Then it happened when it came on so suddenly I was unable to control or stop it. I know you have already solved this mystery; I sneezed so hard it scared me. Even after that, I still had no idea what was happening or why?

No one was with me to tell me it was ok everyone sneezes. It was a while longer before I was able to explain in full detail what was happening then Joel told me all about what sneezing was all about! After that, I wasn't afraid my face was going to come off or something strange was going to happen to my head! I'm happy to say everything is still intact at least that's what they tell me!

After I had the surgery, I was put on 100mgs of Zoloft. I asked why I didn't feel like I had any symptoms of depression. I was told it can happen over time; this pill would protect me from any mental or emotional problems or changes that could happen through the healing process.

So I decided I better take it just incase they're right. Up until the surgery I thought of myself as easy going, I didn't have a temper unless I was pushed, even then it was not that much of a temper. t not long after the surgery, I found myself becoming angry over sometimes the simplest of things and I temporarily lost one of my greatest gifts, patience.

To make things even worse my temper, led to using language I would never have used before! Every time I lost my temper and used bad language, I felt so bad I cried at times. But it didn't stop me from doing it again. Now I see why I was put on Zoloft! I don't remember how long it took before it became effective. I was just so thankful when the day came that I no longer had a temper to deal with!

After around two years, I was taken off of it and have felt fine since. It did help calm me down more than I realized at the time and it was only temporary. Don't think twice if it's suggested you don't have to stay on any type of pill like Zoloft, it will just help you get through a rough transitional period! To make things even worse my temper, led to using language I would never have used before!

Every time I lost my temper and used bad language, I felt so bad I cried at times. But it didn't stop me from doing it again. Now I see why I was put on Zoloft! I don't remember how long it took before it became effective. I was just so thankful when the day came that I no longer had a temper to deal with! After around two years, I was taken off of it and have felt fine since.

It did help calm me down more than I realized at the time and it was only temporary. Don't think twice if it's suggested you don't have to stay on any type of pill like Zoloft, it will just help you get through a rough transitional period!

The one problem I still had two years later was memory retention. I couldn't retain any information for more than a few minutes. I happened to have an appointment to be checked for a carpal tunnel and the doctor noticed right away of the problem with my memory and asked me a few questions. I told him about the brain surgery which everyone thought accounted for memory problems.

Well, it's normal within a period of time after the surgery but not a few years after. He said if you want, I could set you up with a therapist for six weeks. I said that would be great! The first time I saw the therapist, he gave me a test. He handed me a paper that had the alphabet scattered on it, each letter circled. He said just draw a line and connect each letter in order.

He was also timing me. It looked easy enough. I got through maybe a quarter of the letters before I severely slowed down. At this point, they could have been written in a different language. I had to start at "a" every time even the shapes of the letters weren't making any sense to me. I couldn't hide my frustration. Then add shame to it, I was in tears.

How could I not know the order of the alphabet? I was typing questions on my phone since the surgery. I was reading everyday. Why did it take me that long to realize how serious this problem was? My therapist knew how I felt; he was very compassionate and patient. He helped me finish then moved me forward by saying he had some games he knew would help spark my brain into working again.

Once I heard that comment, he had my full attention. He told me the names of the games, 4 in a row, reversi, word find, and mahjongg. He said you can play other games that are similar just make sure they have a rating of 4.3 or higher. I had my tablet and cell phone with me so we started downloading all of them except for mahjong.

I had been playing that one for several years it had always been a favorite of mine. So I made time each day to play each of these games for just a few minutes every other hour or so. Nevertheless, you know the first thing I had to do was to test what the therapist said. Would I get a pain in my head if I were to overdo it? Well I had to test it and yes, he was very correct!

I had a few sharp pains, so I stopped, closed my eyes, and rested! After that, I made sure I didn't overdo it again! The third week I went in and after a few minutes of catching up, I was told I would be given a few more tests, different from the original ones. He said this will determine if you'll need more sessions. If you do we'll be ready to continue.

Again timing me, he gave me several papers to do one after another. I was surprised by how easy they were. I was quickly finished when he said he would go into another room to check them. A few minutes he came back into the room and said he had good and bad news.

The good news is your memory level is at the same point mine is, you did everything just as I asked you. The bad news is you don't have to come back for the last three sessions unless you're bored. Awesome! I had to ask him if these games were for patients who had some type of brain trauma or for anyone. He said they're for anyone, people don't realize they can have fun playing these games and at the same time, their brain is being sparked waking up parts of the brain that have been somewhat dormant!!

I thanked him for all of his help. I still play these games, not every day but often enough to keep my brain from getting lazy! This next story is about a true miracle I was blessed with, one that I will happily tell it until I take my last breath. I hope once you've read my story and you find yourself having a need, you'll want to experience the same thing I have.

Blessed with a miracle...

The pain clinic then extended an invitation to speak with multiple groups

One of the first things I want to tell you to remember is, "Nothing is impossible"! I don't care how many doctors tell you the same thing, anyone that has faith in the Lord, a strong drive, a strong mind, and the desire to have a better life will go as far as they want. I've seen a cancer patient close to dying, healed by the grace of God. No one knows our body better than the one who created it.

Therefore taking our problems to Him, He can repair our health issues immediately. I've been on cloud nine since the first of December 2017 because of a tremendous change that was made by the greatest one in my life, my Lord and Savior. Sometimes unexpectedly, we can go from living a full life to being diagnosed with an illness that changes our quality of life overnight.

It happens to people of all ages every day. But if you've never experienced anything this life-changing, or cared for someone suffering, you wouldn't understand how traumatic it can be. When a true miracle happens, so many people, even Christians want to make one excuse after another because they can't believe it. Seriously, miracles happen every day, unfortunately, the eyes and hearts are blind.

They chalk it up to being lucky. Some people have no idea of how to fathom a true miracle. They still find it so hard to even believe what they can see with their own eyes. I told one person who just didn't want to believe God had the time to heal anyone today. So I had to remind him when Jesus walked this earth, He healed many!!

Gave sight to a blind man, healed a deaf man, healed the lame, and raised a man from the dead, there were countless miracles! Well, He is still alive today and miracles are abundant throughout the world! I am a born again Christian, I'm not perfect, I am a sinner. "Miracles happen so the works of God can be displayed before everyone".

I'm sharing this with everyone to bring praise and glory to God. Those that have never seen me will understand God's power in healing. You are as deserving of a miracle as anyone. By sharing my story, you will recognize which road in life The Lord will guide you on. Once you begin your very first step, He will never leave you.

He wants us to be healthy and happy so we can spread the news about His love for us and to witness to as many people as possible so they will one day live in paradise with Him. He doesn't want anyone lost! Miracles remained in the Bible from thousands of years ago; so that they can be seen every day everywhere, just look around you! But when one happens to you personally, it is life-changing!!

I've been through a lot in my life, the spine surgeries, a total hysterectomy, eye surgeries, to the brain surgery due to a meningioma tumor. That is just a "few" I have mentioned and all have been done in the past 10 years. When I was "finally" diagnosed with fibromyalgia in 2012, I was relieved and at the same time crushed.

I was relieved because someone finally figured it out, crushed because I only heard of it once or twice. I knew whatever I had, I've had all my life, but it was referred to as growing pains when I was young, doctors would say it will pass but it never did. Once this kicked into high gear in 2012, I felt like I was on my deathbed.

The pain was tremendous, I couldn't walk I felt like I had been hit by a tractor-trailer as if I was dying. The first set of meds I was put on took the edge off dramatically, but I couldn't breathe! It turns out I was allergic to the meds. Then I went right back downhill at a high rate of speed. I ended up having to start with a pain clinic because my doctor didn't want to write a drug regularly as strong as I needed.

I thought I was in very bad shape but looking back, nothing compared to the shape I was in November 2017. At this point, I couldn't walk; I needed a walker. I could see myself in a wheelchair. My knees would grind so bad and crack, the pain was unreal, it was like nothing was separating the kneecap anymore.

The muscles in the backs of my calves felt like rocks, every time I took a step it felt like the muscles were having strong spasms and would stretch as hard as they could. I can't express how angry I was. I felt like I was nothing more than a doorstop! I guess I can honestly say I hit rock bottom, physically, mentally, and emotionally.

One thing I've learned is you will know when you have hit rock bottom because you will experience something life-changing. I had experienced a life-changing event once before but it was not nothing I could compare notes to. Another thing, looking back the one thing I kept telling others is if you have the faith of a mustard seed, you can move mountains.

I even carry a tiny zip lock bag with mustard seeds to show anyone I am talking to so they can see how very tiny they are. After it was all said and done, who didn't have the faith of that mustard seed? Me! That's right I didn't believed in what I preached! One night, I was so severely depressed, the pain was taking over, and another pain med was no longer working.

I'll be in a wheelchair next then in a personal care home somewhere, why? I've always witnessed to people, I've tried to be everything you wanted me to be, and I've asked to grow in your word to be close to you. Of all the times over the years, I thought I hit as rock bottom, but this was the first time I ever actually made it there! I kept talking sharing everything from the deepest part of my heart, asking why Father why.

Look at me, I'm unable to do anything for you, My Father, Jesus Christ, you gave your life for me. Sacrificed your blood for me, now I ask you to please wash my body with your precious blood, heal my body of this disease so I can live my life and be available to do anything you need me to do for you. I refuse to live this way anymore, heal my body in your holy name Jesus Christ, I pray in your precious name, Amen.

I not only pictured His blood flowing over my entire body, it felt like a warm honey consistency, I felt the warmth of it completely covering me, starting at the top of my head and it flowed so slowly over my entire body not missing a single spot. I don't even remember or know how I got to bed that night. It was one of the best nights I slept in a long time. The next morning, December first when I woke up, I always just sat on the side of the bed because I would have fallen with the first step from the pain.

Sitting on the bed, I felt pressure on my back. It felt like a hand larger than my entire back was pushing me. I immediately tried to lie back down but at the same time, an angels hand pushed me right off of the bed! I took two immediate steps and stopped. I stopped because I was walking; walking pain-free, I had zero pain in my entire body!

My knees were as smooth as silk, no more grinding, popping, or cracking, I was pain-free! I immediately started crying, thanking my Father in heaven for such an awesome blessing. But what I thought about right away is He healed me because He needs me. Just as I need Him. After that experience, I said a prayer I told Him I would not pray for anything for myself.

He opened my eyes that day, he knows what I need before I do, I am in the best hands possible!! I prayed Father I love you so much, appreciate what you have done for me. With this being said Father All I have to ask is what can I do for you today?

The feeling I had when I realized how awesome the team is that I'm a part of…wow, it's the only team, a winning team!! Since that day, I have thanked Him thousands of times over. I humbly share my story because why enjoy one of the greatest blessings, a miracle and not share it. God wants us to share these miracles with anyone we can. It helps to open our eyes to Him, to draw us closer to him. After that prayer, He gave me someone to talk with or to help every single day!

One thing I forgot to do was to call the pain clinic to tell them I didn't need fentylal patches or the pills anymore. The woman said you can't just stop taking those pills or the patch. You would have to go into a drug rehab, you could go into convulsions. I shared my miracle story with her and said this happened two weeks ago. She then asked you have had no withdrawal symptoms at all.

She mentioned a few I said no, not a one. She said this is impossible I can't understand, how this can be happening, it makes no sense! I shared my frame of mind and my prayer with her and she said you have blown my mind. You hear about things like this but never meet anyone who can tell their story. She was so happy!

To bring light to this message, no matter what a doctor says when you have a close relationship with your Lord and Savior anything is possible. We can't blame Him for our life not being what we think it should be, all He wants is for us to love and accept Him, to believe in His words, to have the Faith of that beautiful tiny mustard seed.

By believing, we'll be able to move every mountain in our path! Trust me; you will never hear a doctor complain about hearing your story and seeing you completely healed. All they want is for you to be well, any doctor would appreciate help from the Master and mine did! I was invited to speak one month before all of the groups there.

The woman I spoke with said we usually only have companies do this but we think your story would love to be heard. I said it would be an honor. She said the only thing is companies bring in gifts for everyone, I said it's not a problem I already know what I'll make and bring in with me. I said I'll send you a picture of what I've been making, she loved it and so did everyone else! Here are a few pictures of what I made and took with me! I enjoyed making these so much!! Everyone loved these key rings!!

Spiritual strength
is
greater than physical strength!

Key Rings

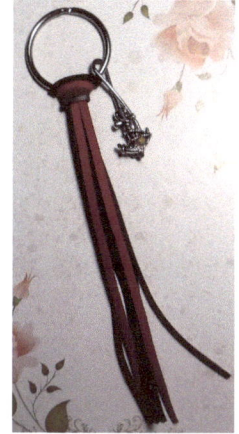
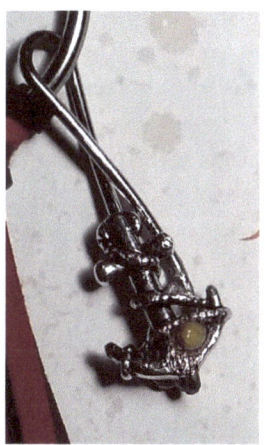

There are 2 chains on the string key rings

to add the mustard see jar and other charms

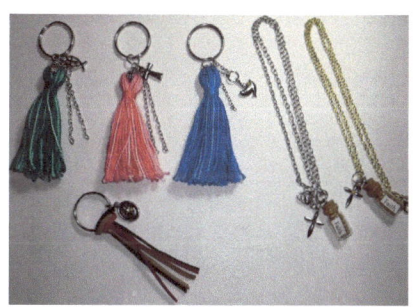
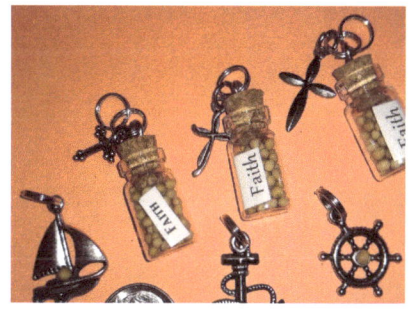
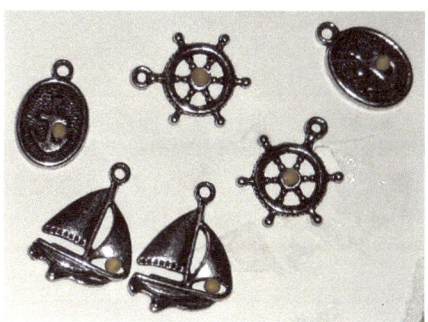

Important questions and answers...

The following question and answer pages have the best case and the worst-case scenarios about meningioma tumors. The last case is more common, we feel we need to give you as much information to make sound decisions concerning your situation. We have also included a list of questions you might want to ask your doctor and surgeon.

1. What is a meningioma brain tumor?

- A meningioma is a tumor that forms on the membranes that cover the brain and spinal cord just inside the skull. Specifically, the tumor forms on the three layers of membranes that are called meninges. These tumors are often very slow-growing. As many as 90% are benign (not cancerous). Most meningioma tumors occur in the brain but they can also grow on parts of the spinal cord.

2. What might cause a meningioma tumor?

- Doctors are not 100% sure what causes brain tumors, but most will agree that a change in an alteration in chromosome 22 (tumor suppression) is the most common abnormality in meningiomas. Also, people that have a genetic disorder called neurofibromatosis type 2 (NF2) are more likely to develop meningiomas. People with malignant meningiomas, a higher percent have mutations in NF2.

- Studies show that patients who received radiation to the head for other conditions are at higher risk for developing meningiomas later in life. There is a correlation between hormones and meningiomas.

3. What is neurofibromatosis?

- Neurofibromatosis is a genetic disorder that causes tumors to form on nerve tissue. These tumors can develop anywhere in your nervous system, including your brain, spinal cord, and nerves. ... The tumors are usually noncancerous (benign) but sometimes can become cancerous (malignant). Symptoms are often mild.

4. What is neurofibromatosis type 2?

- Neurofibromatosis type 2 (NF2) is a hereditary condition most commonly associated with bilateral vestibular schwannomas, also known as acoustic neuromas. These are benign (noncancerous) tumors that occur on the nerves for balance and hearing leading to the inner ear.

5. How common is Neurofibromatosis?

- Neurofibromatosis also is known as NF, is a genetic disorder that affects 1 in every 3,000 people. There are three types of NF: NF1, NF2, and schwannomatosis. Neurofibromatosis type 2 (NF2) is much less common than NF1, affecting about 1 in 25,000 people worldwide.

6. What warning signs and/or symptoms would I have if I have a meningioma turmor?

- These are possible symptoms that can change as the tumor grows. It can be different, depending on the type, location, size, and stage of the tumor. Some people have no symptoms at all. Others will have any number of symptoms that can be mild, headaches, vision, and changes. More severe symptoms would be seizures, personality changes and excessive periods of sleeping, weakness in your arms or legs, trouble thinking clearly, loss of smell, nausea to mention a few.

7. Is there more than one type of seizure I could have?

- There are several types of seizures possible with a meningioma tumor. A lesser type of seizure would be called a;

- A.) Convulsive seizure. It would start where you would suddenly stop responding; stare for a few seconds, then imitate chewing motions and smacking the lips. Shaking movements could be isolated to one arm or part of your face. You would then start walking almost like you were drunk. You would walk into walls or furniture and could fall. It usually only lasts a minute or two then takes a few minutes before you're feeling somewhat normal, It common to remember exactly what happened during that time also.

- B.) Grand Mal seizure is a more severe type of seizure. With this type of seizure, your body would stiffen and your muscles would have jerking movements; a person could even bite their tongue, causing bleeding. It is unlikely you will remember this type of seizure because of going into a coma state.

8. How would I know if I had a seizure?

- Seizures can come on very suddenly. Some of the signs would be jerking movements of your arms and legs, the inability to speak, you would babble. You could even experience bladder loss and could pass out. Seizures can last anywhere from 30 seconds to several minutes.

9. What type of doctor or specialist would I see for a meningioma?

- You would be sent to a Neurologist/Neurosurgeon for a diagnosis of a meningioma.

10. To diagnose a meningioma tumor what types of tests would be run?

- It is extremely rare to diagnose a meningioma tumor before they start to cause symptoms. If your symptoms show a possible tumor, your doctor would order a brain scan: and an MRI with and without contrast and even a CT scan could be ordered along with blood work. These tests will allow the doctor to locate the meningioma and determine its size. A regular MRI scan is about 30-60 minutes long and cannot identify moving fluid, like blood in arteries. An MRI with a contrast dye makes the bloodstream stand out.

- With that being said, an MRI without contrast is still very useful. The majority of MRI scans are performed without the 'dye' used in the contrast medium.

11. What can I expect if I have to have surgery?

- The surgeon will remove the tumor or as much of it as possible. The location of the meningioma will determine how accessible it is for the surgeon. If it can't be reached through surgery, radiation therapy may be used. Radiation can shrink the tumor and help prevent it from growing any larger.

12. Who is at risk for a meningioma?

- They are most common in people between the ages of 40 – 70, diagnosed more in women than in men. Meningioma tumors are very rare in children with cases accounting for only 1.5 percent of the total.

13. Can a meningioma tumor grow back?

- Meningioma, like any other type of brain tumor, can grow back after treatment. About 95% will grow in the same area as the original tumor. However, meningiomas are less likely to come back than other, more aggressive types of brain tumors.

14. Are meningioma tumors cancerous?

85-90 % of meningiomas and are benign or show no cancer. 10-15 percent is atypical grade? A meningioma is listed into 1 of 4 grades: A grade 1 tumor is slow-growing. 85-90 % of meningiomas and are benign or show no cancer. A grade 2 tumor grows more quickly and is often called atypical meningioma. A grade 3 the malignant tissue has cells that look very different from normal cells. Grade 4 the malignant tissue has cells that look most abnormal and tend to grow quickly.

15. Will I be able to live a normal life having part of or all of a meningioma removed?

- Everyone will go through different types of problems right after surgery. A few of the health issues could be difficulty walking, weakness in an arm or a leg, behavior problems as well as speech problems. You could be in the hospital anywhere from four to ten days. After you would be released to a rehabilitation center to help you with any problems that came about after your surgery. Walking could be difficult but they will want you to walk as much as possible. You will not walk alone until you've shown strength in your legs and the ability to walk stable. You will also be given speech therapy should it be needed as well as memory therapy. As long as you work with your therapists, you'll improve every day!

16. Are meningioma tumors cancerous?

- 10-15 percent is atypical or malignant (cancerous).

17. What is the tumor's grade?

- A grade I tumor is slow-growing. 85-90 % of meningiomas are benign tumors.

- A grade II tumor grows more quickly and is often called atypical meningioma.

- A grade III tumor will grow and spread very quickly. 85-90 % of meningiomas are benign tumors. It is often called an anaplastic or malignant meningioma.

17. Do you recommend a website that has a support group and reading material that would help me understand more about my condition and how to move ahead?

- The last page of this book has a list of multiple websites to help you find anything you need to know about meningiomas.

18. Should I get a second opinion?

- You should always consider a second opinion if possible.

19. Do you feel a local support group for people with brain tumors would be beneficial?

- Support groups can be very helpful in any health situation. Your family doctor would be able to give you information on a group in your area.

Meningioma Brain Tumor Questions to ask your neurosurgeon or doctor when a treatment plan has been decided.

1. What are my treatment options?
2. What clinical trials are available for me? Where are they located, and how do I find out more about them?
3. How many brain tumors do you treat each year?
4. What treatment plan do you recommend? Why?
5. What is the goal of each treatment? Is it to eliminate the tumor, help me feel better, or both?
6. Would any of these treatment options keep me from participating in a clinical trial in the future?
7. When should I start treatment?
8. Who will be part of my health care team, and what does each member do?
9. What are the possible side effects of each treatment, both in the short term and the long term?
10. How will this treatment affect my daily life? Will I be able to work, exercise, and perform my usual activities?
11. Could this treatment affect my sex life? If so, how and for how long?
12. Could this treatment affect my ability to become pregnant or have children? If so, should I talk with a fertility specialist before treatment begins?

13. What level of care giving will I need during treatment and recovery?

14. If I have questions or problems, who should I c

What type of surgery will I have?

1. How long will the operation take?

2. How long will I be in the hospital?

3. Can you describe what my recovery from surgery will be like?

4. Who should I contact about any side effects I experience after I'm home?

5. What are the possible long-term effects of having this surgery?

Questions to ask about having radiation therapy or therapies using medications…

1. What type of treatment is recommended?
2. What is the goal of this treatment?
3. How long will it take to give this treatment?
4. What side effects can I expect during treatment?
5. Who should I contact about any side effects I experience? And how soon?
6. What are the possible long-term effects of having this treatment?
7. What can be done to relieve the side effects?

Questions to ask about planning follow-up care

1. What is the chance that the tumor will come back? Should I watch for specific signs or symptoms?
2. What long-term side effects or late effects are possible based on the treatment I received?
3. After treatment, what follow-up tests will I need, and how often will I need them?

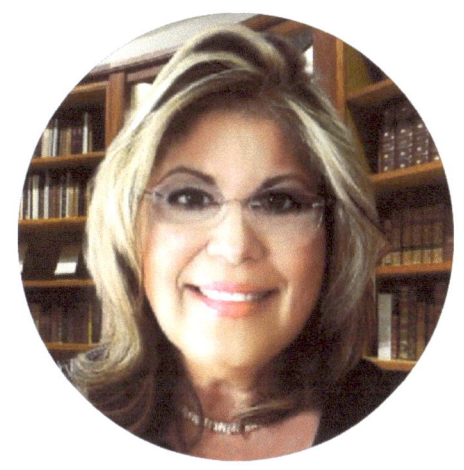

Sharon Getz Brubaker

I was born on December 19, 1958, in Johnstown, Pennsylvania. I have 2 sons, Stephen Brubaker and Benjamin Brubaker. Both have blessed me with grandchildren. Stephen has one son, Tyler, Benjamin and his beautiful wife Andrea have three children; Andrew, Julia, and Luke.

Julia blessed me with a great-grandson on December 19, 2018, on my birthday! His name is King and he is the light of my life! I try to learn something new every day because when I'm done learning, I'm done living. I have no problem with criticism. When the right person takes the time to criticize me that tells me they see me as worth their time, being open-minded and willing to grow.

I am an idealist at heart with the ability to sometimes see and understand what others cannot. I learned at an early age to trust my gut feelings. I always believe everything happens for a reason. When possible, I try to deal with and then file every problem as it arrives. You don't know what's right around the corner.

Forgiveness is a top priority; I don't hold grudges or judge people. Faith is my highest virtue, followed by patience, which I'm thankful for because of the lessons I've learned in my life. I love helping people in any way possible, the more I'm able to do for and give to others the better I feel about myself. I love to make people laugh; it can change their whole day as well as mine!

I always try to keep a positive outlook on life. I hate negativity. I'll do whatever I can to prove someone wrong when they say it can't be done; my first thought is to watch me! I thank God at the end of every day especially if it was a lesson-learned day. He knows every need in my life, I talk with Him often. I don't ask for anything. He has always taken care of my needs before I even knew I was in need.

Every morning when I wake up I thank Him for the day, tell Him how much I love Him then say, Father what can I do for you today? He hears me every time I've always had at least one sometimes multiple things He sends to me to do. Finally, I always tell people I know but don't get to see often how much I love them, how much they mean to me, what an inspiration they have been. Because too often close friends and family have become so used to every day, nothing ever changes. You, forget to tell one another how much you love respect and appreciated one another. If you were to lose someone close to you, it would never be the same. Don't wait until it's too late; tell everyone who has been your best friend, how much they mean to you!

Written In Christian Love,

Sharon Brubaker

Positive thoughts for every day…

When you set your mind to something, anything is possible!

If what you are facing right now doesn't challenge you, you will never grow from it!

Put aside the hurt, forget the pain, but don't forget the lesson it has taught you!

The person you see in the mirror is the one person that can change your life!

The mission ahead of you is never greater than the strength inside of you!

Meningioma Website Links

I wanted to include several meningioma websites to help you find additional answers and information. Using your favorite internet search engine, type any question(s) you have about meningiomas, doors will open to multiple websites. I just want to give you a couple of very informative sites to start with and read. Please remember, your neurosurgeon will answer any questions you have.

1. The American Brain Tumor Association (ABTA): https://www.abta.org

I had the honor of writing my story on this website. The following link will be the page it was posted to. https://www.abta.org/testimonials/meningioma-tumor-a-wake-up-call/

This is something most people don't realize, websites like ABTA loves to hear from people who have been treated for meningiomas. They're happy to post your story because we are educated by those who have also walked the road we are about to start or are already on. Any time you are on a webpage and they mention they would love to hear your story, write to them, you'll be happy you shared it as well as the people will read it!

2. My Meningioma Facebook Group I started at the time the book is published! Please look us up, join and share the page!! I'm looking forward to as many people that we can get!! It's called Meningioma…It's all in your head!!

https://www.facebook.com/groups/391255315220399

3. Johns Hopkins' Meningioma Center is part of the Comprehensive Brain Tumor Center, one of the largest brain tumor centers in the world, with expertise in diagnosing and treating all types of brain tumors, including meningiomas. This information will help you find other meningioma centers in the area you live in. This link I'm sharing is titled The Most Common Brain Tumor: 5 Things You Should Know. It talks about how meningiomas can grow in different places in the skull. It is beautifully written for everyone to understand. It had photos (drawings) showing where the tumors usually are found, talks about different symptoms depending on the location.

https://www.hopkinsmedicine.org/health/wellness-and-prevention/the-most-common-brain-tumor-5-things-you-should-know

4. The Mayo Clinic:

https://www.mayoclinic.org/diseases-conditions/meningioma/symptoms-causes/syc-20355643

5. The Cleveland Clinic:

https://my.clevelandclinic.org/health/diseases/17858-meningioma

6. American Association of Neurological Surgeons:

https://www.aans.org/en/Patients/Neurosurgical-Conditions-and-Treatments/Meningiomas

7. Vanderbilt Skull Base Center is located in Tennessee and is an Advanced Skull Base Tumor Care Center. They specialize in brain tumors!!

https://choose.vanderbilthealth.com/skullbase/?gclid=CjwKCAiA7t3yBRADEiwA4GFlI0HXvw7CI6-boIRHb5jzOzEeJorVLjeXNnutcFfysbosmK_qOHZSMhoCpJAQAvD_BwE

The Mustard seed Parable

The Mustard Seed Parable and Inspirational Thoughts

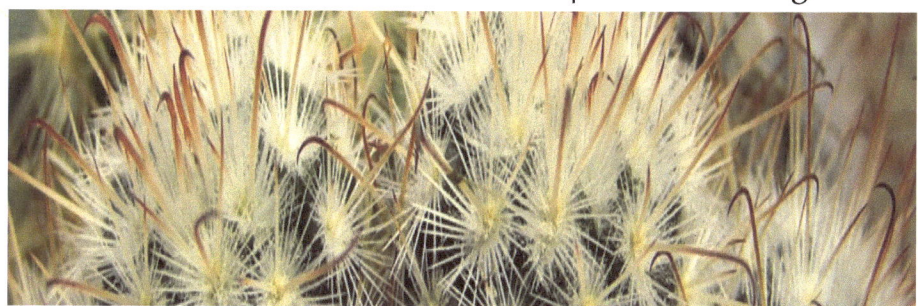

Having the Faith of a mustard seed you will be able to move every mountain on your journey with the Lords help!

The story of the mustard seed!

Stories like this one are referred to as a "Parable". The mustard seed parable is one of the shorter ones Jesus told. It's written in the books of;

Matthew 13:21-32 He set another parable before them, saying, "The Kingdom of Heaven is like a grain of mustard seed, which a man took, and sowed in his field; which indeed is smaller than all seeds. But when it is grown, it is greater than the herbs, and becomes a tree, so that the birds of the air come and lodge in its branches."

Mark 4:30-32 (NIV); What shall we say the kingdom of God is like, or what parable shall we use to describe it? It is like a mustard seed, which is the smallest seed you plant in the ground. Yet when planted, it grows and becomes the largest of all garden plants, with such big branches that the birds of the air can perch in its shade

Luke 13:18-19 reads He said, "What is the Kingdom of God like? To what shall I compare it? It is like a grain of mustard seed, which a man took, and put in his own garden. It grew, and became a large tree, and the birds of the sky lodged in its branches."

The illustration describes the growth and expansion of God's kingdom on earth, the growth of the Christian Church. How the Church began in a small province of the Roman Empire and it grew larger than the mightiest empire on earth.

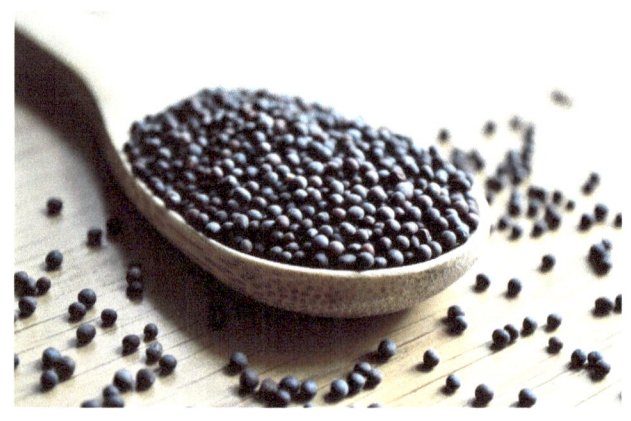

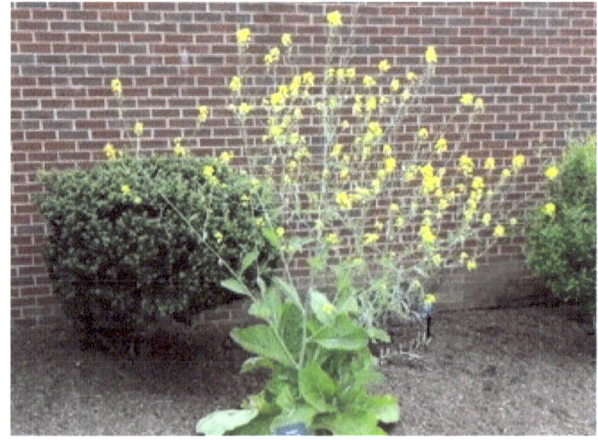

Another time when Jesus used the mustard seed in an illustration was when he was in Caesarea Philippi. Jesus wasn't with His disciples when a man asked them to heal his son, possessed by a demon. The disciples were unable to heal the son. Jesus arrived and ordered the demon to leave the boy (Matthew 17.14-21).

After Jesus expelled the demon, disciples asked him why they couldn't heal the man's son. Jesus replied that they had too little faith. He then said if you had faith the size of a mustard seed, you could say to a mountain, "Move from here to there" and the mountain would move (Matthew 17.21 ESV). Jesus' point to them was that nothing is impossible with sufficient faith, even when that amount of faith is as small as a tiny mustard seed.

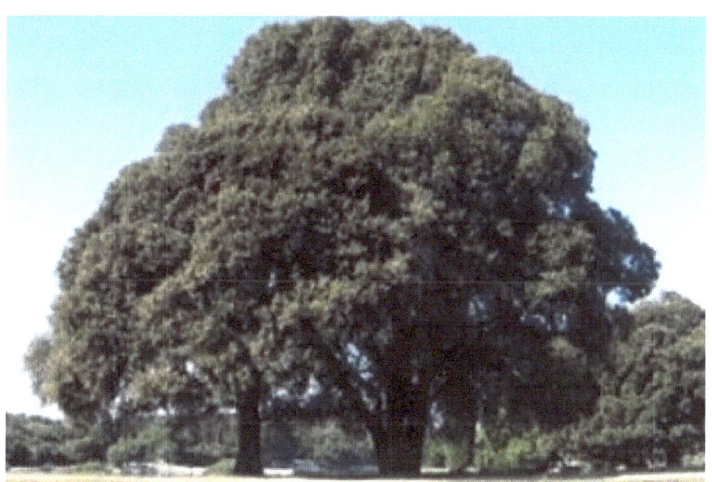

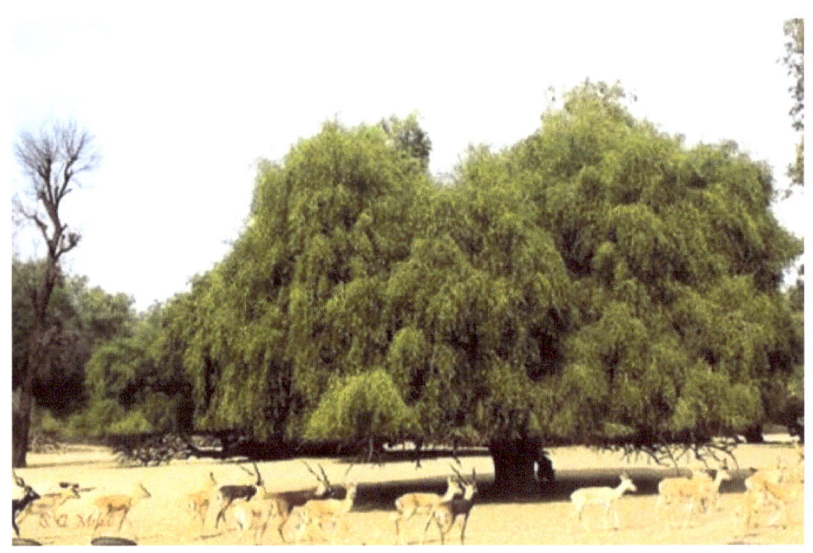

The plant referred to the black mustard seed a large annual plant that can grow anywhere from up 9 to 20 feet tall, growing from a immensely small seed. The size of this same seed also used to refer to faith in Matthew 17:20 and Luke 17:6.

The Mustard Seed Parable and Inspirational Thoughts

This parable actually has three parts: a picture part, the reality part, and the point trying to be made. The picture part is how this tiny seed grows into a large plant, the reality part is, it's the kingdom of God, and the point to be made is the growth of the kingdom of Heaven starts out small and grows taking over the world!

The mustard seed plant doesn't attract birds, it has been said the birds on the plant represent all of the people, the sinners who have accepted the Lord as their personal savior. Jesus gave his life for us so that we would be able to enter the Kingdom of Heaven and be with Him. Don't think when he was dying on the cross God didn't cry, the pain was so great.

But He gave His son as a sacrifice for all of us out of the purest love we'll ever know. No matter how you look at it our Lord has as much time for you and I that we have for Him. He created us for a reason. One day we will have the honor of walking, talking and spending eternity with Him. The Lord loved using parables. He felt they made it very easy for anyone to understand what He was trying to say and teach.

Spiritual strength is by far greater than physical strength!

Believe in the Lord and the words He has written for you!

Trust in your Lord and Savior; Love Him with all your heart!

When you are feeling down...there is only one way to look Up!!

Important notes to keep!

Important notes to keep!

Pre-surgery notes.

Day after surgery notes.

Day of surgery Diary

Day of surgery Diary

Day of surgery Diary

The first few days of healing after surgery

The first few days of healing after surgery

Notes

Notes

www.ingramcontent.com/pod-product-compliance
Lightning Source LLC
Chambersburg PA
CBHW051153220526
45473CB00003B/764